Asperg

The Simplified Guide to High-Functioning Autism Spectrum Disorder and to Raising an Organized Child

Serah Y. Meirre

Table of Contents

ISBN: 978-1-63750-055-2

Introduction

Several parents have found the facts they need about high-functioning Asperger syndrome, in this indispensable guide.

This Complete Guide on Asperger's Syndrome is the definitive handbook for anyone affected by Asperger's syndrome (AS). It brings together a wealth of information on all aspects of the syndrome for children through to adults.

The chapters examine causes and indications of the syndrome; the diagnosis and its effect on the individual; the perception of emotions in self and others; understanding AS and ASD, including friendships; long-term relationships; teasing, bullying and mental health issues; etc... Essential reading for families and individuals affected by AS as well as teachers, professionals and employers coming in contact with people with AS, this book should be on the bookshelf of anyone who needs to know or is interested in this complex condition.

When you meet anyone who has Asperger's symptoms, you may not notice immediately, the victim is just as smart as other people, but has more trouble with interpersonal skills; he/she also will come with an obsessive concentration on one subject, or perform the same actions over and over.

Doctors used to think about Asperger as another severe condition; however, in 2013, the latest edition of the typical publication that mental health experts use, called *The Diagnostic and Statistical Manual of Mental Disorders (DSM-5),* change how Asperger syndrome has been categorized.

Today, Asperger's symptoms are technically not just a diagnosis alone; it is now part of the broader category called *autism spectrum disorder (ASD).* This band of related mental medical issues stocks some symptoms. However, lots of individuals still use the word Asperger; precisely, the condition is what doctors call a *"high-functioning" kind of ASD*; this implies that the symptoms are less severe than other types of autism spectrum disorders.

The DSM-5 also contains a new analysis, called *social pragmatic communication disorder*, which includes some symptoms that overlap with Asperger; doctors utilize it to describe individuals who have trouble speaking and writing but have usual cleverness.

Chapter 1

Symptoms of Asperger Syndrome

Asperger syndrome symptoms start early in a victim's life, and if you are a mother or father of a youngster that has this syndrome symptom, you might observe that he can't make visual contact. You may even find out that your son or daughter seems uncomfortable in sociable situations and doesn't know very well what to state or how to respond when someone foretells him.

He might miss sociable cues that are apparent to other people, like body gestures or expressions on people's encounters; *for example, he might not recognize that when someone crosses his hands and scowls, he's upset.* Another signal is that your son or daughter may show few emotions in that he or she might not smile when happy or giggle at a tale, or might speak in a set robotic kind of way.

If your son or daughter gets the condition, he might discuss about himself and different subjects with a lot of intensity over and over again, especially on a topic that he's thinking about, he could also make the same motions again and again; he may even dislike change, for example, he might eat the same food for breakfast or have trouble moving from one class to another during the college day.

How to Get a Diagnosis

If you notice the symptoms of Asperger syndrome in your son or daughter, see your pediatrician. He can send you to a mental health expert who specializes in ASDs, like one of:

- Psychologist: He diagnoses and solve problems with feelings and behavior.
- Pediatric neurologist: He detects conditions of the mind.
- Developmental pediatrician: He is an expert in conversation and vocabulary issues and other developmental problems.

Psychiatrist: He has experience in mental health issues and can prescribe medication to take care of them.

The problem is often treated with a team approach, which means you may see several doctors for your son or daughter's care.

The physician will ask questions about your son or daughter's behavior, including:

- When did you first notice them?
- When did your son or daughter first figure out how to speak, and exactly how does he communicate?
- Is he cantered on any topics or activities?
- Will he have friends, and exactly how does he connect to others?
- Then he'll observe your son or daughter in various situations to see firsthand how he communicates and behaves.

Treatment

Every child differs, so there isn't any one-size-fits-all approach. Your physician may need to get one of these few therapies to find one which works.

Treatments range from:

- *Sociable skills training*: In organizations or one-on-one classes, therapists teach your son or daughter how to connect to others and go inappropriate town ways. Public skills tend to be best discovered by modeling after typical behavior.

- *Speech-language therapy*: This can help improve your kid's communication skills; for instance, he'll understand how to employ a traditional up-and-down design when he talks rather than flat firmness. He'll also get lessons about how to maintain a two-way discussion and understand cultural cues like hand gestures and attention contact.

- *Cognitive-behavioral therapy (CBT)*: It can help your son or daughter change his thought process, so he can better control his feelings and repeated behaviors. He'll be capable of getting a deal with on things such as outbursts, meltdowns, and obsessions.

- *Parent education and training*: You'll learn lots of the same techniques your son or daughter is taught, and that means you could work on public skills with him at home. Some family members also visit a counselor to help them offer the difficulties of coping with someone with Asperger's.

- *Applied behavior analysis*: It's a method that stimulates positive interpersonal and communication skills in your son or daughter -- and discourages behavior you'd like not to see. The therapist use compliment or other "positive encouragement" to get results.

- *Medication*: There aren't any drugs approved by the FDA that individually treat Asperger's or autism spectrum disorders. Some medicines, though, can help with related symptoms like *depressive disorder and anxiety*. Your physician may prescribe a few of these:

- Selective serotonin reuptake inhibitors (SSRIs)

- Antipsychotic drugs

- Stimulant medicines.

Chapter 2

Understanding the Differences between Asperger Syndrome and Autism

Distinguishing between Asperger Syndrome and autism is challenging. Ongoing research on autism-spectrum disorder shows that this is continually changing; that which was accepted two decades ago has been revaluated and reclassified, which is likely that the views we've today will be significantly different in two decades.

Asperger Symptoms is a comparatively "new" disorder, having been described in 1944 by Hans Asperger on the motivation of Leo Kanner's description of autism. Asperger's work continued to be untranslated for several decades; so that it was not before the 1980s when the broader English-speaking world become familiar with the term. Through the entire 1990s, Asperger's became a standardized medical diagnosis.

Over time, Asperger Syndrome has been classified and reclassified as either being within the autism spectrum or as a completely separate disorder. Inside the autism spectrum disorder, Asperger was often significant to be a "milder" of "high-functioning" form. While children and adults with Asperger's do talk about common symptoms, some key variations make an instance for delineation.

Variations between Asperger and Autism

Many people who have autism will score below-average on intelligence assessments, such as IQ. People that have Asperger's, on the other hand, predominantly rating on par with or more than their peers; frequently, they have superior IQ ratings.

Generally, people who have Asperger do not have problems with speech impairments or inabilities that often characterize people that have an autism spectrum disorder. While there could be difficulty in understanding the subtitles of talk (like idioms, jokes or sarcasm), people who have Asperger's possess the capability to speak and annunciate obviously.

Furthermore, autism spectrum disorders are usually spotted in children before they reach school-age. It is because the symptoms (and their intensity) present much sooner than those of Asperger's. This is because Asperger attacks sociality and communication; it quickly will go undetected until an affected child encounters troubles in school.

Differences between Asperger and Autism

Asperger is also named "milder" and "high-functioning" form of autism; there can be an incorrect assumption that these children and adults live comfortable lives than people that have other developmental disorders; this isn't always the situation; children and adults with Asperger's have numerous challenges, a lot of the problem comes in shared misperceptions of sociable situations and conversation. People who have Asperger's often do not "get" jokes, puns or sarcasm. They might not read body gestures correctly. They could be emotionless or may be unreactive to a situation. It is because of this, people who have Asperger's may induce a kind-of self-isolation because they "don't easily fit into"; likewise, peers could find them uncomfortable or even rude. Those that experience this kind of cultural isolation are vulnerable to panic and depression; they might be puzzled or frustrated, which leads to anger and volatility.

Chapter 3

How common are Asperger Symptoms?

Autism, including Asperger symptoms, is much more prevalent than most people think. There remain 700,000 autistic people in the United Kingdom - that's more than 1 in 100. People who have Asperger syndrome result from all nationalities and social, religious, and sociable backgrounds, though it appears to affect more men than women.

How do people who have Asperger syndrome see the world?

Some individuals with Asperger symptoms say the world feels mind-boggling, which can cause them considerable anxiety. Specifically, understanding and associating with other folks, getting involved in everyday family activities, college, work, and cultural life can be harder. Other folks may know intuitively how to connect and disconnect, yet can also battle with building rapport with people who have Asperger syndrome. People who have Asperger symptoms may question why they may be 'different' and feel their public variations mean people don’t understand them.

Autistic patients, including people that have Asperger syndrome, often do not 'look' disabled, some parents of autistic children say that other folks think the youngster is naughty. We are educating the general public about autism through our excessive amount of information campaigns.

Diagnosis

A medical diagnosis, usually includes a multi-disciplinary diagnostic team, and often, a conversation and vocabulary therapist, pediatrician, psychiatrist, and psychologist, this is because Asperger's symptoms vary broadly from individual to individual, hence, making and analysis can be difficult. It is diagnosed later in children than autism, and sometimes troubles might not be recognized and diagnosed until adulthood.

The advantages of a diagnosis

Some people visit a formal analysis as an unhelpful label,

but for many obtaining a timely and thorough assessment, medical diagnosis may be helpful because:

- It helps people who have Asperger symptoms (and their own families, companions, employers, colleagues, educators, and friends) to comprehend why they could experience specific problems and what they can do about them.
- It allows visitors to gain access to services and support.
- Discover more about diagnosis and ways to get one.

How Asperger symptoms are diagnosed

The characteristics of Asperger syndrome change from one person to some other, however, for a diagnosis to be produced, a person will most likely be assessed as having had persistent problems with social communication and social interaction and restricted and repetitive patterns of behaviors, activities or interests since early childhood, to the extent these "limit and impair everyday functioning."

Learning much more about diagnostic requirements and the triad of impairments theory.

Persistent problems with interpersonal communication and sociable interaction

Social Communication

Autistic patients, including people that have Asperger syndrome, have a problem with interpreting both verbal and nonverbal language like gestures or modulation of voice. Many employ a real knowledge of vocabulary and think people always mean precisely what they say. They could find it hard to use or understand:

- Facial expressions.
- Modulation of voice.
- Jokes and sarcasm.
- Vagueness.
- Abstract concepts.

People who have Asperger syndrome will often have excellent vocabulary skills; however, they may still think it is hard to comprehend the anticipations of others within discussions, perhaps repeating what your partner has just said (this is named echolalia) or speaking at size about their passions.

It often really helps to speak in a definite, consistent way and also to give people time for them to process what has been taught to them.

Social Interaction

People who have Asperger syndrome frequently have difficulty 'reading' other folks - recognizing or understanding others' emotions and motives - and expressing their feelings. This may make it very difficult to allow them to navigate the cultural world. They could:

- Look insensitive.
- Look for time only when overloaded by other folks

not seek comfort from other people.

- May behave 'strangely' or in ways regarded as socially inappropriate.

- They may think it is hard to create friendships. Some may choose to interact with other folks and socialize but may be uncertain about how to start it.
- Reading more about communication and public interaction, sociable isolation, and general skills.
- Limited and repetitive patterns of behaviors, activities or interests

Repeated Behaviour and Routines

The world can appear as though "precarious and confusing spot" to people who have Asperger syndrome, who often prefer to have a daily routine indeed. They could also always want to eat similar food for breakfast every time.

The usage of rules may also be significant. It might be difficult for you to have a different method of something after they have been trained the 'right' way to do it. They might not be more comfortable with the thought of change, but might be able to deal better if indeed they can plan changes.

Highly-Focused Interests

Many people who have Asperger symptoms have extreme and highly-focused interests, often from a reasonably early age. These can transform as time passes or be lifelong and can be anything from artwork or music to trains or computer systems.

Many routes their interest in learning, paid work, volunteering, or other meaningful occupation. People who have Asperger symptoms often state that the quest for such passions is fundamental with their wellbeing and joy.

Sensory Sensitivity

People who have Asperger syndrome could also experience over- or under-sensitivity to noises, touch, preferences, smells, light, colors, temperatures, or pain. For instance, they could find certain sounds, which other folks ignore or filter, unbearably noisy or distracting. This may cause stress or even physical pain. Or they might be fascinated by lamps or spinning items.

Different titles for autism

Over time, different diagnostic brands have been used, such as autism, autism spectrum disorder (ASD), autism spectrum condition (ASC), classic autism, Kenner autism, pervasive developmental disorder (PDD), high-functioning autism (HFA), Asperger syndrome and Pathological Demand Avoidance (PDA). This reflects the various diagnostic guides and tools used and the different autism profiles offered by individuals.

Due to recent and upcoming changes to the primary diagnostic guides, 'autism spectrum disorder' (ASD) is currently likely to end up being the most given diagnostic term; Asperger symptoms remains a good profile for most diagnosticians and experts.

What can cause Asperger syndrome?

The exact reason behind autism (including Asperger syndrome) continues to be investigated; research into causes shows that a mixture of factors, both hereditary and environmental – may be taken into consideration of such development. It isn't the effect of a person's upbringing; their public circumstances, and it is not the problem of the average person with the problem.

Is there a remedy?

There is no 'cure' for Asperger syndrome. However, there's a selection of strategies and methods which people could find to be helpful.

The problematic history of Hans Asperger

Asperger syndrome stocks its name with Hans Asperger, a prominent physique in the first research into autism who worked as a pediatrician in Austria in the 20th century, including before the Nazis. The eight-year investigation into his romantic relationship with the Nazi program was released in 2018, concluding that he aided in their euthanasia program.

This provoked a massive issue among autistic people and their families, particularly those who identify with the word 'Asperger.' We hear carefully to the response to the information so we can continue to ensure the vocabulary we use to spell it out autism reflects the choices of autistic people and their own families.

List of the signs or symptoms of Asperger

Social-behavioral symptoms can start as soon as infancy. Quality differences have emerged in interpersonal development, but these changes are hard to recognize in toddlers and could be related to another condition or not regarded as irregular. Most instances of Asperger's symptoms are identified when the kid is school-aged or old; studies show an average age group at an analysis of 11 years. A number of the symptoms which may be present are:

- Lack of friendly awareness
- Lack of desire for socializing/making friends
- Difficulty making and sustaining friendships
- Failure to infer the thoughts, emotions, or feelings of others
- Either gazing too intently or avoiding eyesight

contact

- Insufficient changing facial manifestation, or use of exaggerated face expressions
- Inadequate use or understanding of gestures
- Lack of ability to perceive non-verbal cues or marketing communications
- Failing to respect interpersonal limitations
- Unusually sensitivity to noises, touch, odors, tastes, or visual stimuli
- Inflexibility and over-adherence to or reliance on routines
- Stereotypical and recurring electric motor patterns such as hand flapping or arm-waving.

Another defining quality of Asperger's symptoms is *the existence of perseverative and obsessive interests in particular topics* (such as cars or trains or higher thin such problems as, floor cleaners), which might be of little interest to others.

These interests are unusually repeated and intense in comparison with other children's interests.

Specific or narrow interests remain the concentrate of the child's interest and conversation regardless of efforts to redirect the child's attention.

Vocabulary development in children with Asperger's symptoms is usually healthy as opposed to other autistic conditions. Children with Asperger's symptoms have regular ratings on assessments for vocabulary function, including vocabulary, syntax, and sentence structure. Some experts believe the existence of healthy vocabulary development distinguishes Asperger's symptoms from high-functioning autism. However, the utilization or software of vocabulary skills is modified in people who have Asperger's symptoms:

Their speech may be disorganized or not highly relevant to the discussion, or they could focus too intently on the defined market (see above) in conversations. The kid may change topics for no apparent reason in the discussion, often so that they can steer the debate toward his / her market.

Changes in tone of voice and speaking (for example, talking too loudly or dramatically, using an invariant shade or incorrect intonation, loud pitch, or speaking too rapidly or too slowly) may also be seen.

Vocabulary may be interpreted literally, and issues can arise with explaining vocabulary in a particular context. There are problems with understanding the subtle use of languages, such as irony or sarcasm.

In college, children with Asperger's symptoms tend to excel with rote learning often required in the first grades. Because they get older, they could have more complications in school because of the character of reading understanding and written projects. Exceptional education support may also be, however, not always necessary.

Sometimes, people who have Asperger disorder have other associated psychiatric conditions or may show behaviors that are typical for differentt states. Some typically standard related terms are the pursuing (but they are not necessarily present):

- Attention deficit hyperactivity disorder (ADHD).
- Anxiety disorder.
- Oppositional defiant disorder or other disruptive behavior disorders.
- Depressive disorder or other feeling disorders

Chapter 4

5 Characteristics of the Person with Asperger's Syndrome

Asperger's Symptoms are one of the disorders that are usually considered high working on the Autism spectrum. People with Asperger's Symptoms, known as ***Aspergians***, have problems with lots of impairments, namely the public, but can also have problems with engineering skills. *For instance, Aspergians have a problem with communication in many ways; they could have accepted guidelines or patterns that are usually very restrictive.*

- **Intellectual or Creative Interest**

Lots of the diagnosed Aspergians will have at least a definite field of intellectual or artistic interest and skill. Americans show exceptional talent in their market and effectively master it later in life. Wolfgang A. Mozart is a superb exemplary case of an actual number with Asperger's-like characteristics. Mozart was incredibly skilled at composing music; he was recognized to write as a kid and continued doing this past due to life. Aspergians may flourish in areas such as photography, web page design, accounting, executive, or data access.

- **Speech Differences**

Speaking distinctions such as insufficient verbal rhythm, monotone pitch, and a peculiar inflection on certain words impact most Aspergian children. Adult Aspergians have the same characteristics because so many do not outgrow it. They are generally struggling to control their voice's quantity according to their surroundings. It isn't uncommon to listen to Asperigans speak loudly in silent places like a host to worship or a library.

- **Delayed Electric motor Development**

Some children with Asperger's Syndrome have postponed development with fine and gross electric motor skills. Children with postponed excellent engine skills may battle to keep a pencil correctly or when grasping items with their fingertips. Delayed gross electrical motor skills can include incapability toss a ball overhand or golf swing on monkey pubs even after a repeated demo. This quality varies broadly and can be observed in both moderate and more severe cases.

- **Poor Public Skills**

For their small fields appealing and a minimal emotional capability, Asperger patient feels isolated through the majority of their childhood years and into adulthood. Asperger patients do make an effort to make friends; however, they tend to be either temporarily successful or ultimately unsuccessful because of the lack of interpersonal skills. In the long run, they sometimes screen too little interest or even attention for the conversations, the viewpoint of individuals they temporarily befriend.

The introduction of Harmful Psychological Problems

The prospect of the development of harmful psychological disorders typically occurs during puberty or immediately after that. The most frequent complications are anxiousness and depression. Regrettably, young Asperger patient has a higher rate of suicide, which may be straight related to stress and anxiety and major depression. The only other demographics with an increased suicide rate for teens is transgender and homosexual individuals.

Positive Characteristics of Several People with Asperger

Most kids, young adults, and adults with Asperger have a couple of positive characteristics that more than make-up for just about any negative ones. One Aspie asserted, "Say thank God I have Asperger!" Let's take a look at only several positive qualities that lots of with Asperger's may have.

Most of them:

- Have the ability to forgive others quickly.
- Are conscientious, reliable, and honest.
- Are enthusiastic and also have a propensity for obsessive research, thus having a broad and deep base of knowledge in subjects appealing is free from prejudice.

- Are intelligent and talented.
- Are less likely to be fickle or bitchy than their neurotypical counterparts.
- Are much more likely than those of the overall populace to pursue a university or college education.
- Aren't inclined to lie to others.
- Aren't inclined to take from others.
- Are not apt to be bullies, people, or public manipulators.
- Aren't motivated by an extreme social drive to invest time with whoever is available.
- Are persistent, so when they collection their minds to something or make a promise, they can usually be trusted to check out through.
- Are improbable to release unprovoked episodes, verbal or elsewhere, are untainted by the judgments that individuals often make regarding

one another's sociable position or public skills.

- Have become accepting of the quirks and idiosyncrasies of others.
- Bring an extremely original perspective to problem-solving.
- It can be selective, choosing honest, genuine, reliable people who share their interests.
- May bring up several interesting facts.
- Can pay attention to people's problems and offer a brand-new perspective, offering fair assessments predicated on the info provided.
- Can recall fine details that others miss.
- They can relax and become themselves without fearing sociable censure.
- Don't assault the reputations of those around them.
- Don't discriminate against anyone predicated on competition, gender, age, or any other surface criteria.

- Don’t force others to surpass demanding sociable expectations.
- Don’t have hidden agendas.
- Don’t play mind games.
- Don’t take benefit of other’s weaknesses.
- Don’t usually recognize hierarchies, and are also unlikely to provide someone superior position simply because see your face is wealthy or has attained a higher status within an organization.
- Have a good work ethic.
- They have a lot of passion when participating in activities they like, which might result in talent for several athletic pursuits.
- Tend to abide by routines.
- Have above-average intelligence.
- Come with an acute sensitivity that facilitates creative talents.

- Have exceptional memories.
- Have extreme endurance.
- Have high integrity.
- Have no fascination with harming others.
- Have several highly developed talents.
- Have skills for going swimming, rowing, running, muscle building, or alternative activities that require suffered physical effort.
- Have ideas that aren't shaped by economic, public, or political influences.
- Judge people predicated on their behavior - not the color of their pores and skin or socioeconomic status.
- Like to spend some time alone and are flawlessly capable of interesting themselves.
- Loathe small talk and trivialities, preferring instead to discuss essential things that will improve their knowledge base.

- Make outstanding employees if in a position to control their speed and work within the solitary or socially supportive environment.

- Focus on detail.

- Adhere to their positions, even when confronted with extreme social pressure.

- tend to become experienced in the technological media necessary for lucrative employment in the "information age group."

- Tend to choose individual sports activities to team sports activities, as there are no social needs plus they can exercise complete control over the experience.

- Develop a pastime in sport or fitness that will probably work at it every day, often for extended periods

- Will not go with the masses if indeed they know that something is wrong.

Chapter 5

Common Traits

Public/Communication Traits

- Despite a desire to have friends, difficulty in initiating or keeping close relationships

- Problems reading nonverbal or public cues or understanding/using sociable rules

- Very socially naïve and consequently are often rooked, turned down, or bullied

- They may direct interpersonal contact (e.g., play is "on the conditions" or never)

- Poor (or intense) eyes contact, atypical use of gestures and smooth or inappropriate face expressions

- One-sided conversations and little ability for "small talk."

- May appear excessively shy or excessively

extroverted

- Unacquainted with others' thoughts, emotions or perceptions leading to inadvertently showing up rude or inconsiderate

- A literal interpretation of communication from others

- Avoidant of public contact or occasions, and could experience heightened nervousness in sociable situations

- Vocabulary is learned and found in "chunks" (e.g., phrases, dialogue from Television shows, etc.)

- Communication is utilized for delivering information or requesting, much less a means of interacting socially

Behavioral Traits

- May respond poorly to changes, sensory stimuli, transitions, insufficient structure, and restrictions

- Repetitive actions (e.g., jumping, rocking, pacing) and talk (i.e., discussing favorite topics, interest)

- Rigid, inflexible and rule-bound behavior
- Inappropriate behavior during interpersonal situation (e.g., speaking too noisy instead of worship)
- Exaggerated psychological response to situations (e.g., tantrums when asked for something that they don't wish to accomplish)
- Superior ability to concentrate on preferred activity or market (e.g., spends hours learning to game to the exclusion of other pastimes)

Cognitive Traits

- Average to superior intelligence
- Detail-oriented method of tasks which might lead to missing the "dilemma."
- May have associated learning disabilities (e.g., nonverbal learning impairment)
- Frequently have high verbal ratings in a cognitive evaluation and low-performance scores

- Difficulty viewing “parts-to-whole” and “whole-to-parts” relationships
- Prefer complex/factual information over abstract

Associated Challenges

- Stress and depression
- Attentional challenges (e.g., moving attention; going to unimportant stimuli)
- Tics or Tourette Syndrome
- Gross and fine electric motor deficits
- Poor organizational skills (e.g., time management and planning, partializing tasks.

Chapter 6

Romantic Relationship for Adults with Asperger's Symptoms and High-Functioning Autism

While an adult with classic autism can happen quite happy with a solitary "monastic" lifestyle, this false with adults who've Asperger's symptoms or high-functioning autism. Clinical experience has determined that most such adolescents and adults would like an enchanting relationship. However, there is undoubtedly remarkably little research examining this facet of autism spectrum disorders (ASDs) or ways to facilitate successful relationships.

We realize that adults with Asperger's symptoms have significant difficulty developing peer relationships and are developmentally delayed in knowing what someone may be thinking or feeling. Typical children do that naturally and also have practiced relationship skills with family and friends for quite some time before applying these capabilities to attain a successful partnership.

Adults with a diagnosis of Asperger's syndrome or high-functioning autism likewise have conspicuously limited social conversational skills or ability to communicate emotions, especially affection. Also, they can come with an extreme sensitivity to particular sensory experiences. Many of these diagnostic characteristics will affect relationship skills throughout childhood, and can eventually limit an adult's ability to accomplish a long-term fruitful relationship.

To achieve a productive relationship, a person must also understand and respect him- or herself. Self-understanding and self-reflection can be especially difficult for individuals with Asperger's symptoms. Self-respect will have been adversely suffering from being rejected, ridiculed, and suffering from peers. Children with Asperger's symptoms are also gullible and susceptible to being given misinformation on relationships by fellow teenagers. This may include cases of being deceived and "setup." For instance, an adolescent with Asperger's syndrome was lonely and desiring a girlfriend. His requests for a date have been consistently rejected. A trendy and attractive girl in his class suggested each of them get a date at the cinema. He was so happy, and the date was progressing well when the lady became embarrassed and confessed that she asked today him and then complete a dare from her friends. He was devastated.

LOVE AND AFFECTION

People who have an autism spectrum disorder have difficulties understanding and expressing feelings, and a feeling that is especially confusing to people who have ASD is love. Typical children and adults enjoy frequent expressions of affection, learn how to express affection to communicate reciprocal feelings of adoration and love, and know when to correct someone's feelings by expressions of affection. A kid or a grown-up with ASD might not seek the same depth and frequency of expressions of love through acts of affection, or recognize that a manifestation of affection is expected in a specific situation and would be enjoyed by your partner. They might be bewildered as to the reasons other people seem to be "obsessed" with expressing love for every other. Someone with an ASD also may be conspicuously immature in his / her expressions of affection and sometimes may perceive these expressions of affection as aversive experiences. *For instance, a hug may be regarded as a distressing squeeze that restricts movement.* The individual may become confused or overwhelmed when likely to demonstrate and revel in relatively modest expressions of affection. I've recently developed a cognitive behavior therapy program for children and adolescents with Asperger's syndrome to clarify the emotion of love and the ways expressing that you want or love someone. This program will soon be evaluated in a study conducted by the University of Queensland in Australia.

Special Interests

Among the diagnostic characteristics of Asperger's symptoms is the introduction of particular interest that is unusual in conditions of its concentrate or strength. In adolescence and early adult years, the focus can be considered a person, that could be interpreted as an average teenage "crush," however the intensity plus some of the associated behaviors may lead to accusations of stalking or harassment. The predisposition to build up a particular interest can have other effects on the introduction of relationship knowledge. Special interests have many functions for individuals with Asperger's syndrome, and one of them is to obtain knowledge to comprehend bewildering areas of their experiences. Teenagers with Asperger's syndrome often are wanting to understand and go through the social and relationship world of their peers, including romantic relationships and sexual encounters, but there may be problems about the way to obtain information on relationships and sexuality.

A teenager with Asperger's syndrome usually has few, if any, friends with whom they might discuss and become informed about related topics such as romantic or sexual feelings and the codes of sexual behavior.

Unfortunately, the foundation of information on relationships for adolescents with Asperger's syndrome can be pornography for males and tv "soap operas" for females. The individual with Asperger's syndrome can assume that the actions in pornographic material give a script of what things to say or do on a date, but this misunderstanding may lead to being charged with a sexual offense. The charges tend to be for sexually inappropriate behavior rather than sexually abusive or sexually violent behavior.

Adolescent women with Asperger's syndrome could use tv programs and films as source material to find out about relationships, and neglect to recognize that the actions and themes aren't a precise portrayal of how to attain and keep maintaining a relationship in life.

Medical experience indicates that previously socially excluded and unpopular teen girls with Asperger's syndrome have, following the physical changes that occur at puberty, become flattered by the interest of teenage boys. Because of her naivety, the adolescent girl might not recognize that the eye is sexual rather than a means for the boy to enjoy her personality, company, or conversation. She may haven't any female friends to accompany her on an initial date, or provide sound advice on dating and the social and sexual codes; consequently, her parents could become worried about her vulnerability to promiscuity, adverse sexual experiences, and date rape.

The Partnership Continuum

There's a relationship continuum from an acquaintance to being truly a partner, people who have Asperger's symptoms can have problems at each stage on the continuum. To advance along the partnership continuum from a pal to a boyfriend or girlfriend, a teenager or an adult with Asperger's syndrome must understand the art of flirting and romance to be able to accurately browse the signals of mutual attraction and understand the dating game. These skills aren't intuitive for individuals with Asperger's syndrome. I am often asked by teenagers and adults with Asperger's syndrome, 'How should I have a girlfriend/boyfriend?' This is not a simple question to answer. Among the difficulties for individuals with Asperger's syndrome is usually to interpret someone's intentions accurately. An act of kindness or compassion can be regarded as a signal of a more profound degree of interest or even more personal than was intended. I possess had to describe to men with Asperger's syndrome that the smile and personal attention of the female person in the cabin crew with an aircraft are signs of courtesy, not indications of the desire to have a relationship.

Regardless of the problems in relationship skills experienced by many people who have Asperger's symptoms, some adults can progress along the partnership continuum and have the ability to experience romantic and, subsequently, intimate personal relationships, even learning to be a lifelong partner. To accomplish such a relationship, both partners at first could have noticed attractive qualities in your partner. What exactly are the characteristics that someone would find attractive in an adult with Asperger's syndrome?

Attractive Qualities of The Person with Asperger's Syndrome

Men with Asperger's symptoms have many qualities that may be appealing to a potential partner. When conducting relationship counseling with one or both partners getting the characteristics or diagnosis of Asperger's syndrome, I often ask the healthy partner, *'What were the qualities that made your lover attractive when you initially met him/her?'*

A lot of women describe their first impressions of their partner with Asperger's syndrome to be a person who is kind, attentive, and socially or emotionally immature. The word "silent, handsome stranger" may be used to describe a person who seems relatively quiet and beautiful. Physical characteristics and attentiveness can make a difference, especially if the girl has misgivings regarding her self-esteem and physical attractiveness. The man's insufficient social and conversational skills can result in his being regarded as the "silent stranger" whose social naivety and immaturity can be transformed by somebody that is an all-natural expert on empathy, socializing, and conversation.

I've noted that lots of the companions of men, and sometimes of women, with Asperger's symptoms, have been at the other end of the friendly and empathy continuum. They may be intuitive experts theoretically of Brain, namely understanding and empathizing with someone else's perspective. These are naturally gifted in the capability to understand the world as experienced by the individual with Asperger's syndrome, a lot more so when compared to a person of average Theory of Mind abilities. They are understanding and sympathetic, plus they guide his or her partner in social situations. Indeed, they are the characteristics of an adult with Asperger's syndrome recognizes that he/she needs and would find desirable in somebody. She or he will actively seek somebody with intuitive social knowledge, which can be considered a social interpreter, is naturally nurturing, is socially able, and is maternal. However, while a culturally insightful and empathic partner may understand the perspective of the individual with Asperger's syndrome, the individual with Asperger's syndrome has considerable difficulty understanding the perspective of his/her typical partner.

The attractiveness of the person with Asperger's syndrome in a potential relationship can be improved by intellectual ability, career prospects, and amount of attentiveness during courtship. Sometimes, however, this attentiveness could be perceived by others as almost obsessive, and what and actions may have been learned from watching Hollywood romantic movies. The individual can be admired for speaking his mind, even if the comments may be regarded as offensive by others, due to his keen sense of social justice and explicit moral beliefs. The fact that he might not be "macho" or desire to spend time with other men at sports or alcohol consumption can also be appealing for a few women. The individual with Asperger's syndrome can be considered a late developer in conditions of relationship experiences, which can also be a stylish feature. There could be no previous relationship "baggage." I likewise have had a lot of women describe if you ask me how their partner with Asperger's syndrome resembled their father. Using a parent with the signs of Asperger's syndrome may have contributed to their selection of partners as a grown-up.

What exactly are the characteristics that men find attractive in a female with Asperger's symptoms? The features can be like that which a woman finds attractive in a guy with Asperger's symptoms, especially the amount of attentiveness. The woman's social immaturity may be attractive to those men who've natural protective and compassionate qualities. There may be an appreciation of her physical attractiveness and admiration on her behalf, talents, and abilities. Unfortunately, women (and sometimes men) with Asperger's syndrome aren't very proficient at making character judgments or identifying relationship predators. Women with Asperger's syndrome frequently have low self-esteem, which makes a difference in their selection of a partner in a relationship. They could be the victim of varied types of abuse. As you woman with Asperger's told me, 'I set my expectations surprisingly low and consequently gravitated toward abusive people.'

Ways to Improve Romantic Relationship Skills

People who have Asperger's syndrome will demand assistance in relationship skills at each point on the partnership continuum and probably throughout their lives. Children will require guidance from a speech pathologist in the art of conversation and ways to improve friendship skills throughout the institution years from a teacher or psychologist. The introduction of friendship skills must be considered a priority for educational services that support a kid with Asperger's syndrome, as greater maturity and ability in friendship skills will improve self-esteem, reduce incidents be teased or bullied, lay the foundations for adult relationship skills, and encourage teamwork capabilities for successful employment. Adolescents will require accurate information on attraction, the dating game, and sexuality. While these details are shared for typical teenagers, often from friends, parents, classroom programs, and gradual experience, it might not be as common for an adolescent with Asperger's syndrome. Having less peer guidance, group discussion, and practice will inhibit the introduction of relationship skills.

Fortunately, we've programmed on relationships and sexuality created explicitly for adolescents and adults with Asperger's syndrome and advice from fellow teenagers with Asperger's syndrome. Some clinicians and therapists, particularly in Australia, are developing resource material and expertise in teaching relationship skills to adolescents and adults with Asperger's syndrome. The training ranges from enhancing knowledge on dating etiquette and dress sense to learning ways to recognize and prevent sexual predators. A fundamental strategy is to have indeed a socially conscious friend or relative meet a potential date to determine if the person is apparently of good character before creating a relationship.

Young adults will require encouragement and opportunities to make acquaintances and friends. This may include joining a spare time activity or interest group that is associated with a particular interest, such as attending a Star Trek or Dr. Who convention, or it could involve a credit card application of the talent, such as having an all-natural ability with animals and joining an animal protection group. There may be opportunities to socialize at community activities like a local choir or adult education classes. Local Asperger's syndrome organizations for parents established organizations for adults with Asperger's syndrome. This can offer a chance for a specialist to handle the group and offer discussion and guidance in relationships. Such groups can also be a chance for relationships to build up between group members. The partnership that developed between Jerry and Mary, two adults with Asperger's syndrome who met at a support group in LA, has been the main topic of a film and book. Some adults with Asperger's syndrome have used the web and dating agencies to meet people, but relationship predators can also utilize this technique of introduction, and a grown-up with Asperger's syndrome must be familiar with the many risks associated with using this plan.

I've noted that adults who had clear indications of autism in early years as a child (that is, significant vocabulary delay, learning issues, and avoidance of public situations), and who in later youth progressed to an explanation of high-functioning autism, tend to be less motivated to get a long-term romantic relationship. They will be quite happy with solitude and celibacy and having acquaintances rather than friends. A feeling of self-identity and personal value is attained by having a capable profession and being impartial. Temple Grandin is a well-known example. Some adults with Asperger's symptoms also have didn't seek a romantic relationship with someone for legitimate reasons when one considers the characteristics of Asperger's symptoms. Jennifer described her rationale: 'Can I offer with sharing a residence with somebody who might touch my model aircraft collection?' and 'Model airplanes do not decide that they would like to be built by another person who is more appealing or less needy.' Her life will include occasions of extreme personal satisfaction. She says, 'I can assure you that being in love and having special passions are quite a similar feeling.' Devoid of a romantic relationship can be considered a positive choice for a few adults with Asperger's symptoms or high-functioning autism who enjoy going after and are fulfilled by their unique passions, such as animals' photography or a profession in it. They may be content never to be swept away by the ethnic belief that relationship or a long-term romantic relationship is the only path to achieve pleasure.

Areas for Future Research

We realize that adults with Asperger's symptoms have considerable difficulty progressing along the partnership continuum, but we absence research that delivers quantitative and qualitative data on relationship abilities, circumstances, and encounters. There is certainly research on the companionship skills of children with Asperger's symptoms that have been examined, but hardly any research on partner/girlfriend associations and sexuality. *Dr. Isabelle Hénault*, from Montreal, and I have already been performing research on the intimate profile of adults with Asperger's symptoms, and initial results show a different pattern than typical adults in conditions of more inferior body image and fewer intimate experiences, although close interest usually evolves at precisely the same time as with adolescent peers. There can also be considered a more liberal attitude to close variety such as homosexuality and bisexuality, and wealthy dream life and intimate imagery. There could be less concern regarding age group and cultural variations in a romantic relationship.

However, there has to be more research, and the Interactive Autism Network data source may be extremely useful in providing information on passionate relationships for children and adults with Asperger's symptoms and high-functioning autism.

What's Mild Asperger's Syndrome

It is sometimes tough to diagnose mild Asperger's symptoms, which explains why many people aren't diagnosed until these are teenagers or even adults. Often, those who find themselves on the autistic spectrum are dismissed for being only socially uncomfortable when, in most cases, they may be struggling to handle a developmental disorder.

When someone has Asperger's, an excellent mild case from it, which means that they experience difficulty in social skills and communication, also, they experience pain handling sights, preferences, and noises (conscious control).

More complicated situations of autism are usually diagnosed in children ages three and more youthful. Children who've Asperger's, however, primarily a moderate case from it, aren't often diagnosed until down the road because they typically meet most if not absolutely all of their developmental milestones.

A kid with slight Asperger's might not be diagnosed until he begins college and finds it difficult to talk to his instructor and peers. He might have trouble working in the cultural situations that accompany most school-related activities, and he might find it hard to understand instructions that are communicated to him verbally.

Mild Asperger's Symptoms in Adults

Interestingly, what used to be considered "gentle Asperger's symptoms" are no more diagnosed as "Asperger's," but instead as high-functioning autism. Be that as it might, if you recognize the below as things you have observed, you might have been experiencing minor symptoms of high-functioning autism:

- A debilitating degree of difficulty communicating in sociable situations. You might chat a blue streak in what passions you, not recognizing that nobody is thinking about your chosen subject of conversation.

- An inability to produce meaningful relationships. You might have trouble making and keeping friends and co-workers.
- A dependence on repetition and order. If something interrupts your day to day routine, you blow a gasket.
- A passion for a specific topic, and difficulty in communicating with others on any issues in addition to that one. You can talk all night about the annals of the Pontiac without noticing how enough time has exceeded, or how things in your environment had transformed when you were speaking.
- A level of sensitivity to sensory insight, like loud sounds or the flavor of a specific food. A noisy car horn can terrify you.
- Adults don't limit these symptoms; children who are diagnosed as high-functioning can screen the same symptoms.
- Additionally, it is essential to keep in mind that

Asperger's is very individualized, and therefore, not everyone will go through the same symptoms. One individual may haven't any problem along with his regular getting interrupted, while another will not be in a position to function if something in his ordinary is disrupted. One individual may experience problems with his excellent engine skills that triggered a hold off when he discovered to trip a bicycle, while another may haven't any interest in studying activities or topics apart from those he already understands and loves.

Treatment for Mild Asperger's in Adults

There is absolutely no treatment for just about any autism because autism is not a disease. Many who've learned to handle the downsides they have observed using their condition are determined never to seek the formal analysis, which is okay. Others have wanted the medical diagnosis and then do nothing after they knew for sure that these were, in truth, on the spectrum. That's fine, too.

The only time you must do anything for an autism analysis when it inhibits your ability to live life. If you discover it challenging to produce a severe reference to someone, keep down employment, or maintain an adequate liveable space, then it might be necessary that you should seek specialized help to understand how to manage your trouble better.

Internet dating with a Mild Asperger's

When internet dating someone with mild Asperger's (high-functioning autism), it's essential you know just as much as you can about the problem to lessen the number of situations that could lead to a fight more than a miscommunication. Below are a few what to know to get you started truly.

"Aspies" Have A Problem Expressing Their Feelings

If your lover doesn't often let you know how fairly you look, or how much he loves you, it could be difficult never to take offense. Tell him how you feel and clarify to him why it is critical to you that he learns how he can cause you to feel more special. You do not want to feel insecure regularly, and you don't need to when you can help him focus on his communication.

Produce a "safe space" where he seems comfortable discussing these exact things with you. Additionally, it may help take breaks from the discussion, so neither of you feels overwhelmed, particularly if you will need to keep detailing you to make things more transparent for him ultimately.

Aspies Have Trouble Understanding Physical Affection

It may appear strange for you that your lover does not realize why you're kissing him on the cheek or keeping his hands, but it is because he will not recognize that this a physical screen of your love for him. Show him that you will be holding his hands and kissing him because you like him and want to show him this.

If you go set for a hug, you might cause your lover to lash out at you, with him convinced that you want to invade his personal space. This also true if you have never kissed, hugged, or kept hands before. Instead, give your lover a heads-up that you would like to hug him because you feel near to him right now, and have if it's alright to achieve that at that time. This will review superior to if you merely do it now without explanation.

Aspies May Have A Problem Reading Certain Sociable Situations

Aspies have a problem with large gatherings, so if you are thinking about taking him to your loved one's reunion in the summertime, and he backs out, don't take it personally. You will find a wide variety of individual public situations to learn at a celebration or gathering that it could be overwhelming even though you aren't on the spectrum.

If he will decide to opt for you, however, one of the ways you may make the problem go more smoothly for him is to make most of his introductions for him. This will need a few of the pressure from him to comprehend how each individual wants to connect to him and what they expect of him in exchange.

It may help let everyone know beforehand that your lover is on the spectrum, though this may make things worse if indeed they all treat him with child gloves. Instead, it could be easier to describe to your lover the things that individuals may choose to do with him (tremble his hands, hug him) and just why they would like to do these exact things (to state hi, expressing their joy at conference him, etc.). You can even clarify discreetly to your lover the proceedings as it happens.

Aspies may tell you the same tale again and again and forget they ever told you.

CPSIA information can be obtained
at www.ICGtesting.com
Printed in the USA
LVHW080302270821
696253LV00013B/228

9 781637 500552